I0696500

# Finding My Stride:

## A Journey into the Grand Canyon

And the Musings of a Wannabe Backpacker

By BJ Roshone

JP Band Books

*Read the Brand*

Independently published in the United States by Kindle Direct Publishing for JP Brand Books
JP Brand Books, P.O. Box 145, Valentine, Nebraska 69201

JP Brand Books

Cover Design: Bobbie Roshone
Cover Photo: Bobbie Roshone

# Table of Contents

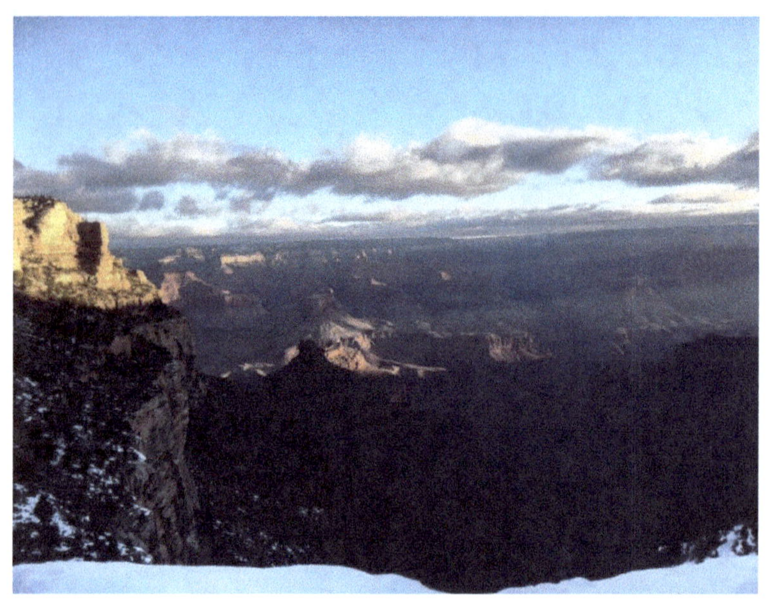

# Grow by the Inch, Die by the Foot:  A Journey into the Grand Canyon

When you first read that heading, it sounds like a story about somebody dying or some other misfortune. It's not that kind of book. This little saying stuck with me during the hike and after when I started writing this blog and it's all thanks to a sign at Havasupai Gardens —now Havasupai Gardens. The sign was behind a wooden rail fence enclosing some desert plants right off the trail. It acted as a warning about how delicate these desert plants were.

Those words would stick with me. It seemed like a metaphor for life in a lot of ways. We grow into the person we are by mere inches, sometimes depending on the person centimeters, but every "foot" we take leads us closer to our demise. And right there it went to that kind of book about dying or some other misfortune.

Let's see if we can bounce back from that. This book, aside from my creepy metaphor about life, is about exploring the natural world around us and growing from its serenity.

This adventure originally appeared on my blog, The Wannabe Backpacker. It's still there if you want to read for free. The blog is on-going, even though I sometimes don't post as much as I should. I finally got around to turning it into a book it would seem. All the events happened to the best of ability to remember. I wrote the original blog nearly a year after I hiked the Grand Canyon and this short little book nearly six years later.

I hope you enjoy this foray into the Grand Canyon.
Find your path.
BJ,
*The Wannabe Backpacker*

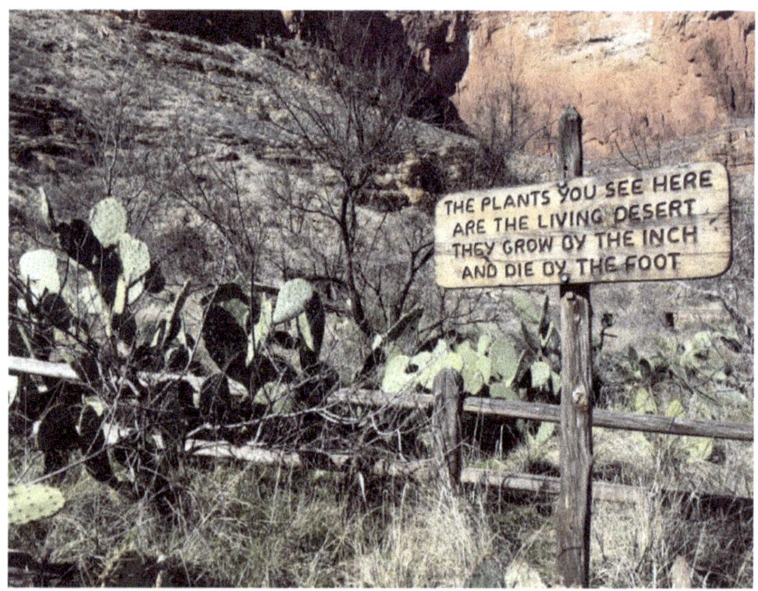


*1. Inspirational sign*

# Dedication

To my family—you are my biggest supporters.
PJ, you are the best writing partner…unless I have to get a
fish. *


(*Sorry inside joke to my sister)

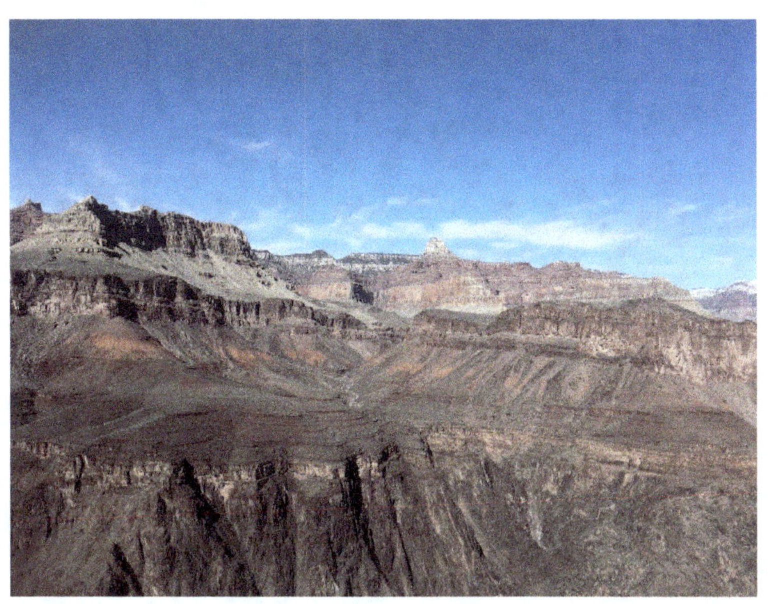

"The glories and the beauties of form, color, and sound unite in the Grand Canyon." – John Wesley

# Havasupai Gardens

*Posted November 23, 2022*

I'm still taking my time writing and working on my blog—
from trips this summer, my float trip on the Current River
in the Ozark National Scenic Riverways and day hikes in
Glacier National Park—lots to write but not a lot of time.

However, this announcement from Grand Canyon National
Park caught my interest and I wanted to post an update
about my first overnight backpacking trip that started this
whole blog! Here is the complete story in one place.

On November 21, 2022, it was announced that the U.S.
Board of Geographic Names voted unanimously (19-0) to
change Indian Gardens to Havasupai Gardens honoring a
formal request from the Havasupai Tribe to the National
Park Service. The National Park Service formally
submitted the request to the U.S. Board of Geographic
Names.

I think the original name, Ha'a Gyoh would have been
more appropriate, but Havasupai Gardens will enlighten
folks to the history of the Havasupai Nation and the history
within Grand Canyon National Park.

I'm still debating if I will go back and change the name in
my original posts; however, in this retelling I did update the
name. Looks like I'll need to plan a return trip to update my
pictures…and paddle the Colorado River.

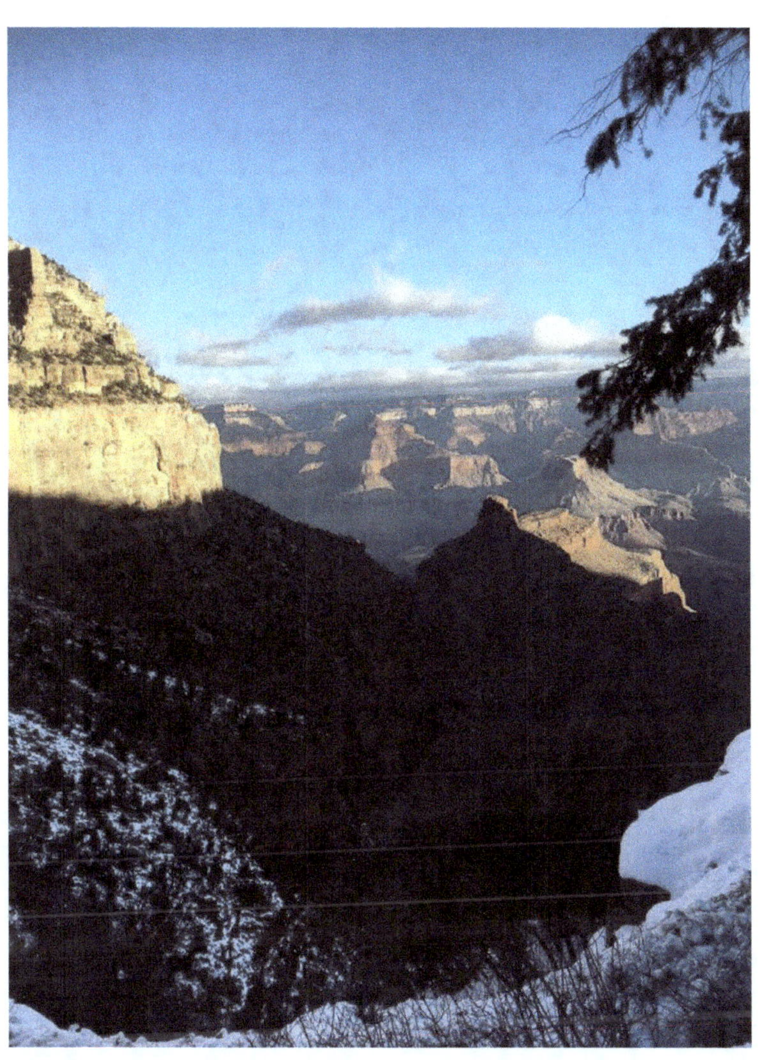

*"The wonders of the Grand Canyon cannot be adequately represented in symbols of speech, nor by speech itself."*

# Part One: Getting Ready
## 2017

February, usually not my ideal time to go for a hike, or even camping for that matter. However, I was at the Grand Canyon! I wanted to experience everything I could while I was there. I was spending two weeks in a classroom for job related training, but the weekend was mine to do what I wanted.

I spent most of the first week in my "off hours" reading over brochures thinking about what I wanted to do on my upcoming weekend. I spent some of that time walking around the dormitory and going to some of the nearby overlooks. I fell in love with the snow-covered desert while I was there.

There were so many options in those brochures. However, I felt like I wouldn't get to really experience the canyon if I did an interpretive program or a "day hike." What I really wanted to do was a rafting trip on the Colorado River but it's kind of hard to do a two-day trip and really experience all the rapids and the amazing geology. I was still planning and re-planning my weekend when the training instructor said something like, "Although, it's wintertime, we did secure some backcountry passes for anyone who wants to do an overnight in the Grand Canyon! The good news is once you get down below it will warm up to the mid-sixties. We have it set up for two groups, a long one that will overnight at Phantom Ranch and a shorter one to Havasupai Gardens."

*"Could I make it down to Phantom Ranch?"* I asked myself while staring down at my feet. I was thinking about blisters, pulled muscles, and sore calves but I could touch

the Colorado River. However, my internal voice piped up with, *"No, your chunky butt would explode. Maybe if you'd lay off the damn cupcakes and ran a mile a day you might make it but you're so out of shape you are a shape."*

My internal voice isn't very nice sometimes.

But it was right, I couldn't do a 17-mile hike overnight and keep up with the group. Not without severely injuring myself in some way. I got lazy over the last year. I started graduate school and slipped back into the bad habits I had in college. Snacking while I was studying, not managing my time well so workouts went the way of the dodo, and stressing myself out because of it, which in turned caused me to eat those delicious cupcakes…

In reality I had only gained twenty pounds (bad but not as bad as my internal voice made it seem) and wasn't as out of shape as I thought. I wouldn't be running marathons, but I could still handle hiking at my pace. After the weekend I realized the weight issue or even the out of shape issue wouldn't have been a problem. It was holding back my stride going down and coming back up that caused my calves to cramp. Although, I'm sure if I had been hitting a stair stepper it wouldn't have hurt as bad.

We had a meeting after that day's training. The instructor and about twenty of us were debating going down. I was still on the fence, but I was determined to go even if it was the shorter hike to Havasupai Gardens and back. While looking at the map and scale, my internal voice said *"Hmm, almost five down and five back spread out over two days, you would probably live through that."*

I concurred, but I wanted to see if anyone else would go. While I felt confident doing it by myself, I wanted at least one other person on the off chance I slipped on the icy parts of the trail. I was starting to get a little worried, everyone else wanted to do the overnight to Phantom Ranch, but once the dust cleared there were three of us willing to do Havasupai Gardens. Two newbie backpackers and an experienced guy.

While I do have a little experience, I still think of myself as a "newbie" or a "wannabe," I know the gear, I understand how to pack the backpack, but I've never spent a weekend, or even a overnight, doing a backpacking trip. The reason I know the information and how to pack the gear is because I'd always planned to backpack the Ozark Trail. I just never got around to doing it before I left for college or leaving for my job in Nebraska.

I'm the queen of procrastination, but I plan like crazy for the "future" trips. I also had to be a familiar with backcountry trips, even though both places I worked at didn't really have established backpacking communities. The Ozark Trail is a big thing where I'm from, but I never really had to deal with it while working for Ozark National Scenic Riverways. Everyone was more interested in the rivers than in taking a backpacking trip.

I also got familiar with ultra-light equipment because I would keep it in my day pack when I was out on a quick hike, just to be on the safe side. I always figured I would be the person that managed to fall over a root, break something, and be stuck outside overnight. I figured with my line of work I should be familiar with the equipment. I even took a backpacking class so I would know the basics.

We had a mini meeting before we raided the gear room. Since I was an EMT and had a little more experience than the other lady going. I would handle the medical gear for the trio and a tent for us girls. I decided to go light on the medical gear just a basic first aid kit with the usual stuff, two Sam Splints, and needed splinting materials.

I remember looking at the gear laid out on the shelves. The first thing I grabbed were crampons and hiking sticks. Since it was winter, the first mile or so down was covered in snow and ice. I'm a klutz, I can fall "upstairs" just as easy as down, and while I'm usually pretty agile on trails and high places I was hedging my bets.

The pack I found wasn't really made for someone of my diminutive size. If I had been thinking I would have grabbed the pack I received as a birthday gift in college after one of my ramblings about becoming a backpacker, and brought it on this trip, it's a perfect fit for me. It also would be great for weekend backpacking trip or ultra-light trip.

I was surprised that nobody really grabbed the mummy bags, which made me happy. Thinking, while during the day the interior of the canyon would be nice and toasty, the night would get cold, I was right on that. Into the pack the mummy bag, mummy bag liner, a couple of dry bags, the two-person tent, and a ground tarp.

I thought about taking a little MSR backpacking stove but since I was already carrying the tent and during our meeting, we were doing are own food I decided to bring stuff that wouldn't require heating and thrifty so I could eat at El Tovar without wincing at the bill later in the week.

Once we had grabbed all the gear, we thought we would need, we huffed and puffed it back to our respective rooms to pack our other essentials. For me that was mainly food and water.

A quick trip to the general store had me stocked up and ready for the overnight. My menu was Bumble Bee tuna snack packs, hard boiled eggs, granola bars, and peanut butter oatmeal bites.

Later, I would regret not bringing the stove. A cooked meal (even if it had been oatmeal) would have been heaven and hot tea would have been lovely on Sunday morning but live and learn. I tossed in a two full sized Snickers bars, a handful of mini 3 Musketeers, electrolyte packets, and New-Skin (the only thing I didn't wind up needing). My special treat: one bottle of Gatorade that I planned on drinking at the bottom of the canyon. I'm weird, I know.

Sidenote on the weird part. I'm a big water drinker…now. I annoy my fiancé, Wade, with how much water I drink and my many bathroom trips. However, I used to not be that way. All through high school I despised water. I lived on Coca-Cola and beef jerky. Why my kidneys didn't fail, or I didn't drop dead I'll never know. But now it's like my body is making up for not drinking water during that time. I think the majority of weight I carried was from water, three full water bottles plus the Gatorade.

Once I was back in the room the packing commenced. After packing all the needed items, I decided to bring my Kindle (I was reading *In a Sunburned Country* at the time), my phone so I could take pictures, and extra socks. I was only going for an overnight and figured my clothes would keep. I finished putting everything in and decided to test the weight.

I had a problem.

The weight wasn't the issue. The pack was made for the Jolly Green Giant. Even after pulling in the straps all the way in, it would still gap on my shoulders pitching the weight back to around my butt/upper thighs.

So, I got creative. I had compression straps from packing two weeks of clothes into a little carry-on. Tweaking the chest strap by adding the compression straps to frame and tying them off on chest strap, it closed the gap It wasn't comfortable, but it was doable. It would shift and bug me, but it wouldn't cause stress to my back and hips at least.

I was ready.

Or at least I thought I was ready.

# Part Two: The Descent

5:00 AM. *Beep. Beep. Beep.* Slam!

I rolled out of bed and showered. We were meeting at six to drive over to the trailhead. I heated up a bowl of oatmeal, had a cup of coffee, and spent five minutes brushing all the plaque off my teeth. I was sacrificing dental cleanliness for contact solution space in my pack so I could wear sunglasses.

Then I fired up my laptop, like I said earlier I was in graduate school. Taking classes online made life easier but it still took (and takes) up a lot of my time. I'm one semester away from having my Master of Science in Secondary Education, come on May 2018! I wanted to see if anyone else had posted in the class discussion so that I wouldn't have to cram everything in on Sunday night. I got lucky and was able to do the two required posts. I would have Sunday night free to relax. Wahoo!

Around ten till six, I put on my favorite pair of hiking pants, t-shirt, long sleeve shirt, and a jacket. Grabbed my stocking cap and pack and headed out the door to wait. It was cold, around 17 degrees. Growing up in southeast Missouri I had a very limited understanding of what cold was until I moved to Nebraska. However, it was a dry cold, so I didn't seem to feel it. There also wasn't the howling wind to contend with like in Nebraska.

I paused to look around, the last few days a couple of mule deer had been wandering around the dormitory grounds and I got a kick out of watching their ears flicker. I hadn't been exposed to mule deer until recently and for some reason, their ears reminded me of goats.

No deer this morning, so I hiked my pack up on my shoulder and meandered down the stairs, the same stairs I would come to loathe on Tuesday.

So far it was shaping up to be a glorious morning. The sun was going to rise around the time we made it to the rim. I was ecstatic as I walked towards the meeting point, the parking lot. The gang was all there.

We had picked up an extra person. She was going to drive us out to the trail head at Bright Angel and hike down with us, then back out before nightfall. After packing the back of the van full of packs, trekking poles, and us we headed out.

The sun was just creeping over the horizon when we pulled up to Bright Angel. I almost needed the crampons and trekking poles to get up to the trailhead. Ice was patchy on the concrete sidewalk and pavement accesses, my klutziness already creating havoc for me. Aside from some slipping I made it to the rim.

The rim of the Grand Canyon is a spectacular place. Standing there at dawn on a cold winter's day? Simply majestic.

It was quiet.

The hustle and bustle of tourist, workers, and sightseers wouldn't show up for another hour or two. Except for the buildings, rails, asphalt, and concrete, when I was standing at the overlook at Bright Angel I could almost image how it was pre-1920. Soon I would be stepping off into a slightly less developed wilderness and I couldn't wait.

We took a few minutes to get our crampons on, trekking poles to the correct length (well I didn't have to do this, sometimes being short is awesome), and taking a few photos. During this time, the sun hit the canyon, creating a beautiful blend of the shades. Reds draining into golds, it was stunning. I could have sat there all morning watching how the colors changed and shadows played with the moving sun.

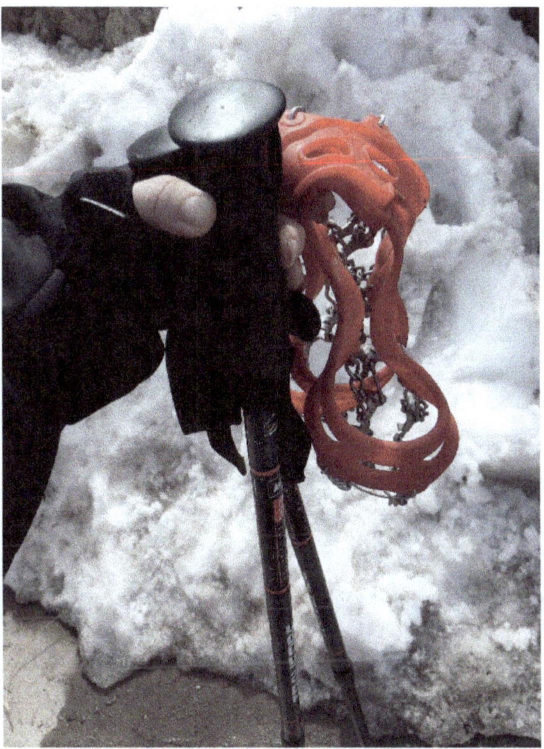

*2. Crampons (ice cleats) and trekking poles are a must.*

I knew though that those colors would be more vibrant and the shadows more dramatic the further down in the canyon. I wanted to see how the sun played on the Colorado River. I wanted to move.

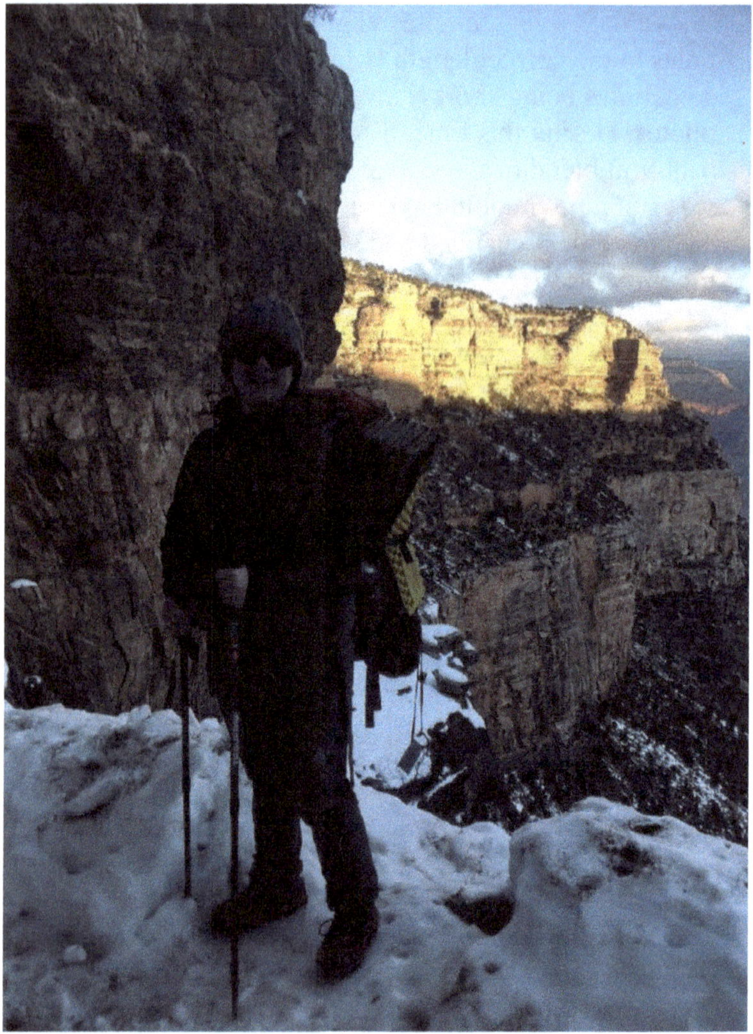

*Figure 3 Author standing on Bright Angel Trail*

I wanted to know how the world was below.

After taking one last group photo clustered around the Bright Angel Trailhead, we began our descent. Since I was the one with medical training, I thought it prudent to be at the back of the group. The most experienced guy would take the lead and everyone else would fall in-between. We stayed within earshot of each other.

Although, as the progression went most of us stayed within two feet of each other. The lead guy would get a little ahead of us and stop and wait for us to catch up. By the end of the trip, I would envy him.

The first mile was cathartic, at least to me. I was back in nature. Hiking down a mountain into a canyon, and I was at peace. The way the trail drops down from Bright Angel we were hiking in the gloaming, predawn, even though we could look out over the canyon and see how the sun was changing the colors.

The switchbacks were tight, cutting back against the side of the canyon. In some places cutting through the rock. Those cuts created beautiful arches to walk under along the way. The further down we got the more meandering the switchbacks would get, with rocks scattered at the perfect interval to sit and talk with other hikers. Or avoid the mule trains.

We were the only ones for a few hours, around nine am we would begin to see a trickle, by eleven there was a flood tourist. But for those first few hours I felt like a character from a novel. I was picturing myself as a great adventurer, like Martha Gellhorn. I get the feeling I was more like Samwise Gamgee or even closer Pippin; I was ready for second breakfast by ten.

I was imaging hot eggs, sausages, tomatoes, and mushrooms; but I had to settle for a hardboiled egg and a granola bar. We had made it to a little rest house just below the snow/ice line. After taking a few moments to drop our packs, pull off the crampons, and use the facilities, we sat down to enjoy the scenic vistas and eat a snack.

I felt good, better than good; this hike was so easy!

My what a big bite of crow I would have to eat a few days later. In that moment though, I was enlivened. I found something I loved; I knew I could take my wannabe status to the next level and become a doer. Heck, I was already doing it and it was amazing!

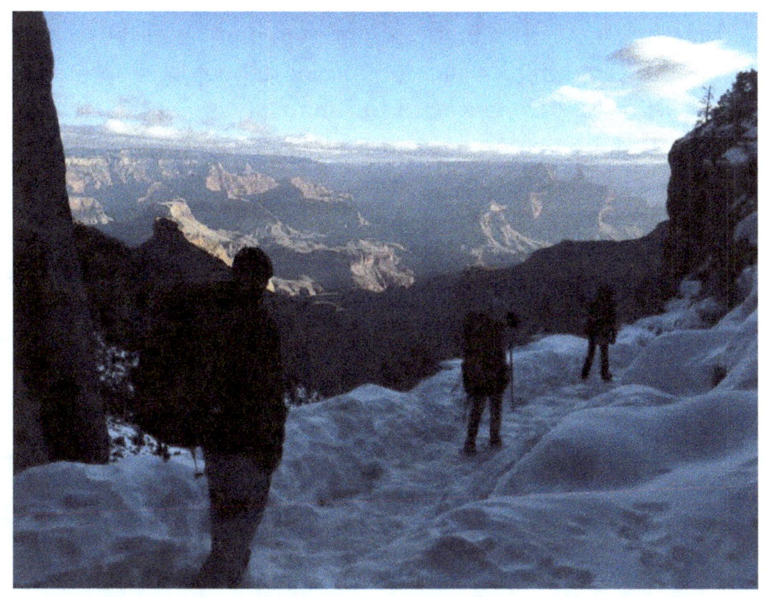



Sitting there looking out over the canyon was mesmerizing; the sun was further up in sky. The temperature jumped up a little higher; enough that my jacket had to go into the pack. I got to watch a mountain blue bird hop from branch to branch on a small bush next to the trail, looking for handouts. Please people, stop feeding the wildlife; they can fend for themselves. To the right a big formation stuck out from the wall of the canyon; it looked just like a battleship.

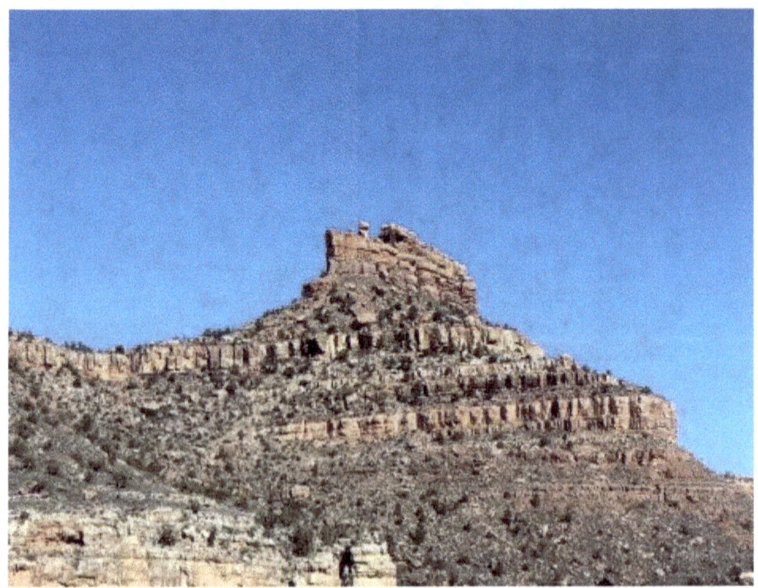

All too soon it was time to start the next leg of the trip. I shouldered my pack and realized I lost some of the stability I had when my jacket was on. I quickly retied it while the others were putting away trash and grabbing their own packs. I realized I wouldn't get the pack tight enough to my shoulders to stop some rubbing.

Even with an ill-fitting pack I was in a good mood; although, the way I had the straps rigged after I took off my jacket the next mile down would have me struggling to keep the pack in place. By the end of the day, my shoulders would be a little raw and sore. But I never lost my enthusiasm.

Each step brought me into a whole new world for me. I grew up in southern Missouri, home of rivers, trees, and world class natural springs. Then I moved to Nebraska, the rolling prairie, the natural crossroads of three different ecosystems, and a river.

Those places I knew and loved; yet I was having to make room in my heart for the desert, for the Grand Canyon. Aside from some of the animals and birds, I didn't know natural aspects of the canyon, only a few of the flowers and plants looked familiar. The geological formations, while breathtaking and fascinating, had me at a loss. I had no knowledge of the names or timeline for the strata lines. I had very limited knowledge of which Native Americans called this place home. I wanted to know more.

Once out of the canyon on Sunday I and another colleague would head to the bookstore; where I spent a small fortune on the books, I would need to answer all the lingering questions I had while hiking. However, I was hiking through one of the most beautiful places on earth; getting all the answers could wait. I had better things to focus on; the canyon itself.

I was walking through a world of ancient rocks. A world of desert plants. A sea of purple cactus, in the low sunny spots. Purple cacti? Why is it purple? Okay so I really can't turn off the endless questions I ask myself. BTW the answer I was given, by a passing park ranger, was because of overheating or stress to the plants in chilly weather.

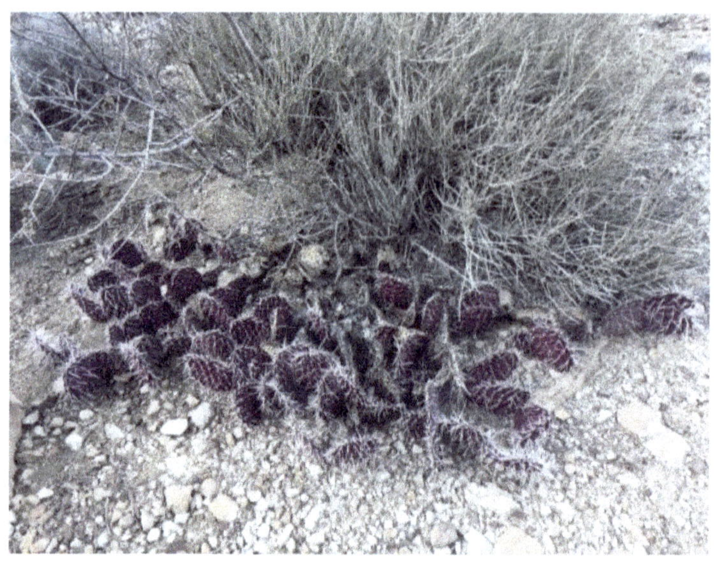

I and the group were starting to get a little tired by this point it was almost noon; the trail hit a series of switchbacks leading down to the bottom. These switchbacks resembled the ones at the top, steep back and forth. At the bottom the trail leveled out, but the damage was done. It was here that my pack would start to bug me the worst and I would realize being at the back and slowing my stride was starting to hurt my legs.

I found this funny; my fiancé, Wade, spends a great deal of time teasing me about being short I am and how I must jog to keep up with most people, especially him. I wonder why all the time I spend jogging hasn't gotten me into shape. The fact that I was outpacing anyone was hysterical. I took a short break letting everyone get ahead of a bit. I ate a 3 Musketeer staring up at how far I had come.
Looking back up at the rim of the Canyon, thinking on the four miles I had trekked. I was proud of myself, and it was only the beginning.

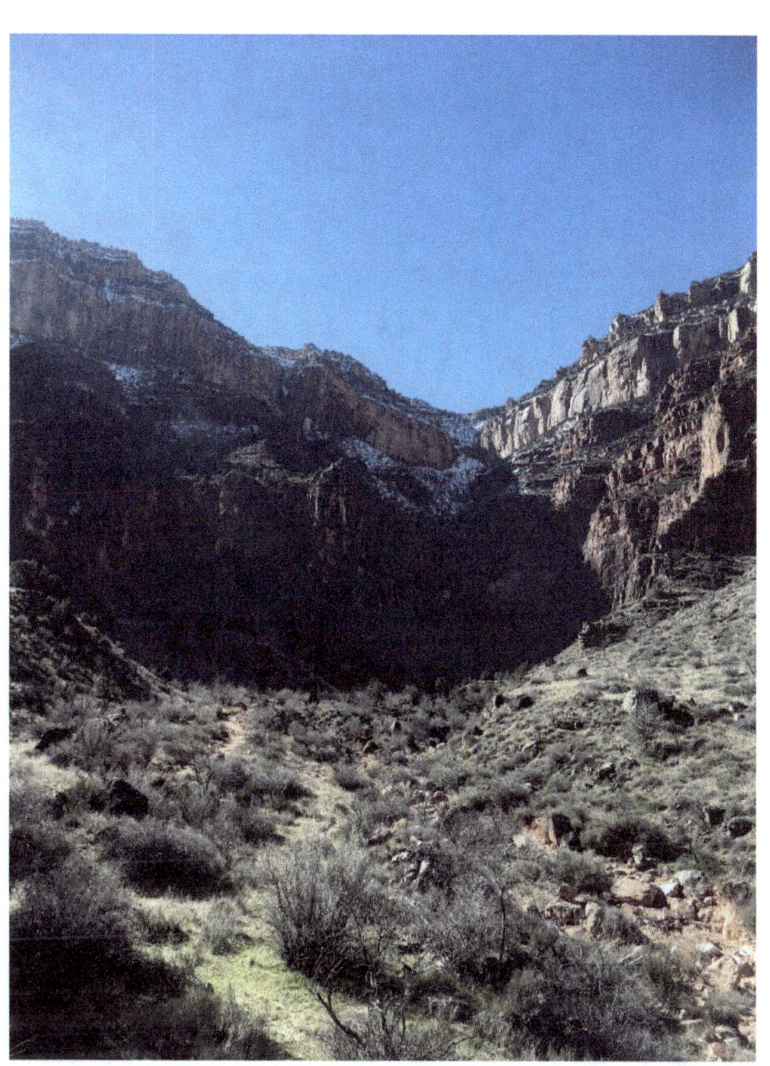

# Part Three: Interlude at Plateau Point

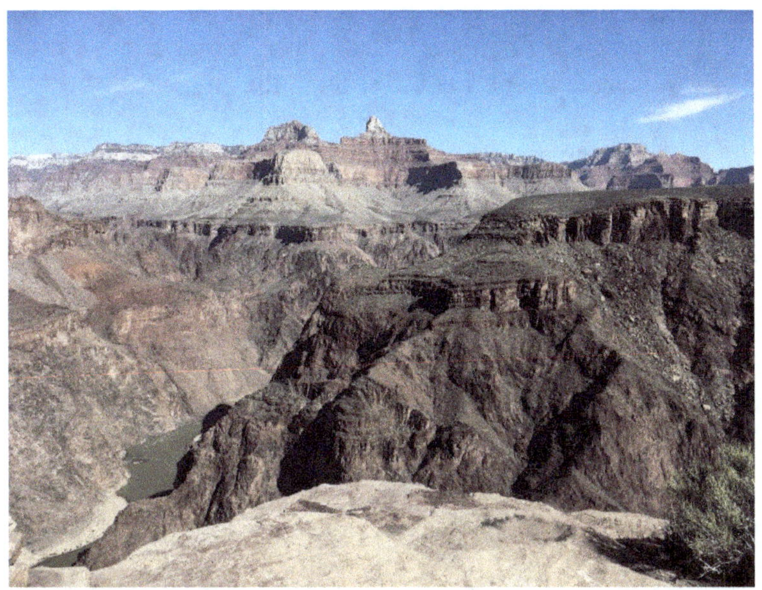

After descending more than 3,000 feet we arrived at Havasupai Gardens, our home for the night. We paused to read a wayside sign about the area and the campground. A little orienting and we found our site.

Havasupai Gardens; is a beautiful place. A perennial creek flows through the campground; I waded into the water even though it was only 60 degrees out, but it felt so good on my sore feet at the end of the day. Cottonwoods and willows lined the small creek framing the ranger lodging/office before flowing into the desert and on to the Colorado. In a lot of ways, it reminded me of an oasis; it was so green compared to the rest of the canyon.

The little ranger cabin/office also housed a little library area for visitors; they could even charge their electronics and find additional information. I collected a few site bulletins about Havasupai Gardens when we stopped in to rest our feet. I really wanted to go work in the Grand Canyon after seeing the backcountry cabin. I could hike every day and finally get rid of those extra pounds caused by cupcakes… and I could still eat the cupcakes.

The campground was so quaint; with little covered shelters that housed a picnic table and old ammo boxes for food storage. Apparently, the rock squirrels, deer mice, and ravens like free food that's tossed to them; who would have guessed? Now, those little critters will just march up to a campsite and steal food lying around; so, put it in the ammo can.

Now from reading the wayside (NPS lingo for guide sign on the edge of the trial) I learned a little bit of the history of the Native Americans in the area, primarily the Havasupai. I had limited knowledge of this and many of the smaller bands that frequented the desert. In college I took several history classes about Plains and Woodlands tribes and for my minor in Folklore I took a Native American Verbal Art class; desert tribes, except for the Navajo and Apache, didn't really come up. I was regretting that now.

Back up on the Rim, while in the NPS bookstore I would find a very interesting book about the Havasupai, their history in the Grand Canyon, history with settlers, and their struggles with the NPS, and other agencies, since the parks creation. It is a worthwhile read, *I Am the Grand Canyon: The Story of the Havasupai People* by Stephen Hirst, for those of you that are interested.

FYI when I'm not hiking, I'm reading, if it's a great book or story about backcountry hiking or historical background I will sing its praises in my blog. Possibly, even base the blog around the book if it features backpacking.

When I sat down and read the book, I was a little heartbroken by what had happened to Gswedva (Big Jim) and Burro's Garden land under the rim and how they were forced off of it to make way for progress. Thinking back to my time in Havasupai Gardens, I could image their heartbreak at having to leave a place they had called home for generations. The sad thing was this didn't happen all that long ago in the grand scheme of things, Burro was forced to leave in 1928.

Many of the other Havasupai would lose their homes on the rim and be regulated to roughly a 500-acre reservation at the bottom of the of an offshoot canyon, along Havasu Creek. Their restriction to the bottom of the canyon occurred in 1882, thirty-seven years before the Grand Canyon became a National Park, and it would take nearly fifty years to move all of the Havasupai from their Rim lands down to the small tract that was only suitable for farming. The Havasupai would augment their harvest with hunting and gathering on the rim in the winter. However, that was no longer allowed and could result in imprisonment if they were found to be supplementing their food storage.

Later in the 1970s the Havasupai would successfully plead their case against strong opposition from NPS, surrounding landowners, and even environmental groups to reclaim lost acreage on the top of the Rim. In 1975, ninety-three years since the small reservation had been established, Congress passed the Grand Canyon National Park Enlargement Act that would return 188,077 acres of both plateau and canyon lands to the Havasupai; enlarging the reservation from its 518 acres.

Sorry for the historical rant; back to the backpacking trip. We got our camp situated, pulled our lunches out, and sat down to plan the rest of our day. After reviewing the map and filling our stomachs; our driver and day hiker was going to return to the top of the rim, the experienced person in the group was going to hike down to the Colorado (I so wanted to do this, but I was a little foot sore and my shoulders were killing me), and the newbies were going to Plateau Point.

Leaving the camping oasis, we had a one-and-a-half-mile hike to Plateau Point, through beautiful open terrain. It was warm, light wind, and sunny. The trail was well maintained and moderately packed with people. Once we got to Plateau Point the visitors had dwindled, only two other people were about, and they left about ten minutes after we got there.

We had the point to ourselves—other than the lizards…

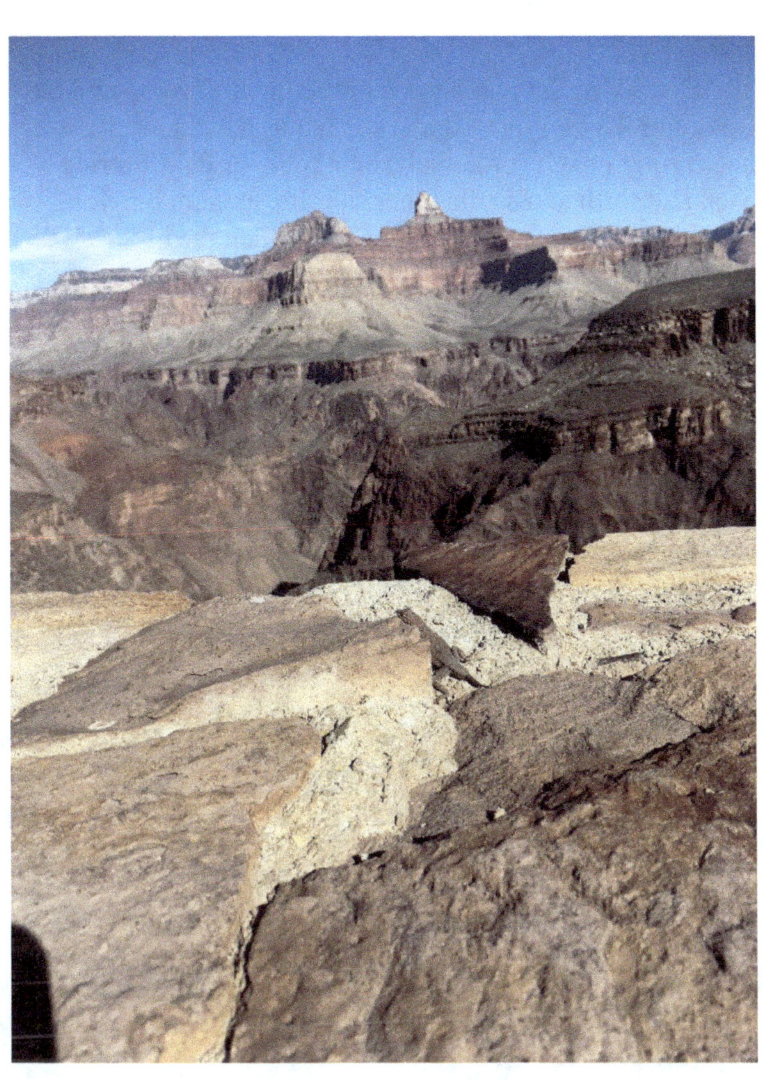

After taking several photos of the Inner Canyon and the Colorado River. I just sat and soaked it in, watching a lizard sun himself (or herself) on a rock, birds' flittering back and forth across the inner rim. It was faint but you could hear the few rapids below and, when the breeze was just right, smell the river. I enjoyed my Gatorade, fruit punch is where it's at, even if it leaves a red mustache. We sat there a good chuck of the afternoon, watching the sun paint the canyon in different colors as it lazily drifted through the sky. All too soon we started our march back to Havasupai Gardens.

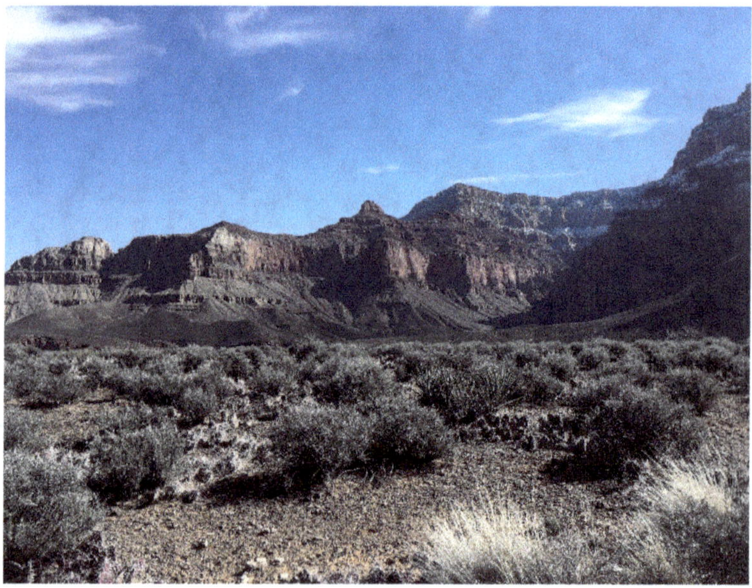

We were just getting back to the rest house at Havasupai Gardens, the sun was just starting to go down, creating a beautiful backdrop to a spectacular day. I was sitting on a bench waiting for my hiking partner to return and to be rejoined by the other guy whom we saw coming back up the Bright Angel Trail from the river. When I was joined by a rather fit you man that was planning on hiking out that night; he had hiked down to the river himself and was making his return.

We got to talking, turns out this was a nearly a monthly trek for him and he loved the canyon. Since the light was fading, we didn't hold him up too long. By the time we had finished talking our fellowship was once again complete. (Did I mention I'm a LOTR fan?) We made our way back to camp for dinner.

It was mid dinner when the park ranger made his rounds checking the permits and visiting with the hikers. He was so cool, and he totally loved his job. He answered several of my questions and recommended nearly half of the books I would buy the next day. Once our meal and conversation had finished, we all wondered off to explore the fading light. I made my way down to the creek and stuck my feet in it again.

Looking at the Rim I was able to see the Watchtower light in the distance, before being overwhelmed with stars. Living in rural (and I mean rural) Nebraska we have excellent night sky conditions. In the Grand Canyon I was blown away. One quick trip to the bathroom and I wound up walking with my hiking partners again. We made one more stop into the ranger cabin, they were looking for something to read. Before returning to camp.

Once the sun went down and we were no longer moving very much it started to get cold. It was an early bedtime for us; we retired to our respective tents. I joyously climbed into my mummy bag and powered up my Kindle. I was reading about Australia in a matter of moments. Bill Bryson has a way with words and after reading about Uluru (Ayers Rock), explaining how it was a sacred place for

Aboriginals' and the eventual British takeover and creating the tourism surrounding it, I had a little moment of connection to how the Native Americans viewed the Grand Canyon, and its colonialization and commercialization is impacting them.

Almost ten o'clock, I was getting sleepy but after drinking nearly a gallon and half of water I needed to make one more trip to the bathroom. It was a chilly walk but just as amazing; I thought the stars had been clear right before we crawled in our tents. I was wrong; everything was so sharp in the sky. I heard an owl hooting on my way back.

I didn't want to leave.

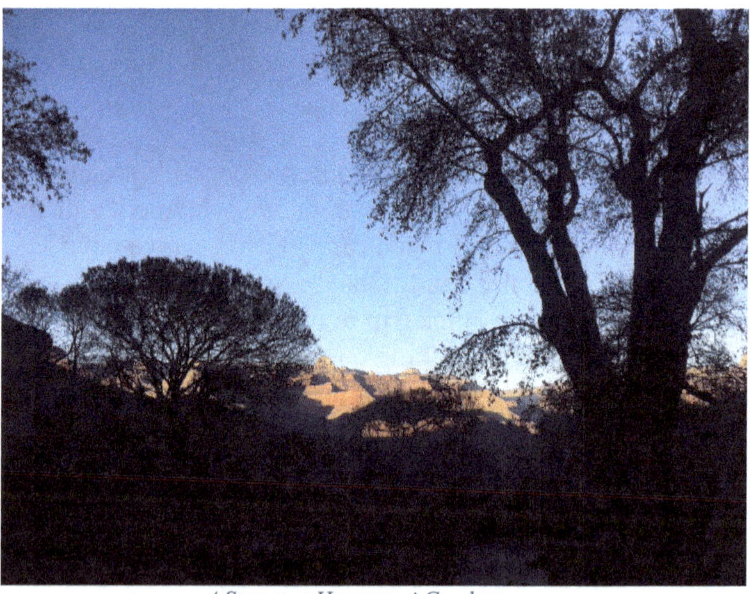
*4 Sunset at Havasupai Gardens*

“Have you camped in the

Grand Canyon?


It’s intents.”


– Anonymous

# Part Four: Return to the Rim

Cold. Blissful cold. If you like that sort of thing. I wanted nothing more than to burrow down deeper into my mummy bag and wait for the sun to rise and warm up the canyon. However, that never seems to work for me when I'm camping.

I'll usually wake up early, if I'm camping with friends, I'll feign sleep. So, I can stay in my tent and read or just relax enjoying the sounds of nature interrupted by the sounds of camp cookware clanking and low voices. I tend to do the same when I'm camping by myself. It's odd when I'm home in civilization I'm a night owl that hates getting up in the morning and I'll sleep in on weekends. Camping, my clock reset's itself, I should camp more often.

This chilly morning in February, I got up with my hiking partner, the other guy had already been up for a while. After the usual morning ablutions, we had breakfast. For me that was one of the hard-boiled eggs and two granola bars. I kept hoping it would magically turn into bacon, tomatoes, fresh bread, and hot tea but alas no magical hobbits were running about cooking breakfast. However, at the time it was filling. Looking back now, I should have had about twice the number of calories. I thought I had planned for the deficit, but I underestimated what I would need for the hike back up.

After breaking camp, I took a few moments to fill up all my water bottles and the now empty Gatorade bottle. We took one last look around Havasupai Gardens s and set off for the return trip up the Rim. My legs were only a little sore and each step seemed to loosen them up.

As we left the green valley of the garden, I looked back towards our resting place, the canyon beyond, and the invisible Colorado River. one day I will come back and explore this place far more. I adjusted the pack, once again better fitting because of the jacket and kept hiking.

We hit the switchbacks right away; for me these, and the switchbacks the last mile up, were the worst. Although, the ones at the bottom, in comparison to the last little bit, were easy. I was enlivened by my experience in the canyon, it was a new day and a new me.

I honestly don't remember as much on the first few switchbacks up. I do remember when at the last two in this section I wanted to find the person that made backpacks (or in the more likely the person that bought them in bulk for the training folks) and find out what his or her problem with short people was, because that pack was getting ridiculous. Did they just not assume short people hiked?

Overall, the trip back up wasn't as exciting as going down; if we had gone on down to Phantom Ranch and back up the South Kaibab Trail or up to the North Rim it would have been more fun for me. However, we were doing a down and back on the Bright Angel Trail. I still loved it, but I had seen most of the views on the way down.

I will say the view heading up was impressive. The Rim a huge wall just towering above you, it's daunting but when you make it to the top it makes you feel invincible. The other reason I don't think I enjoyed it as much was the impressive amount of people that clogged the last two miles of trail.

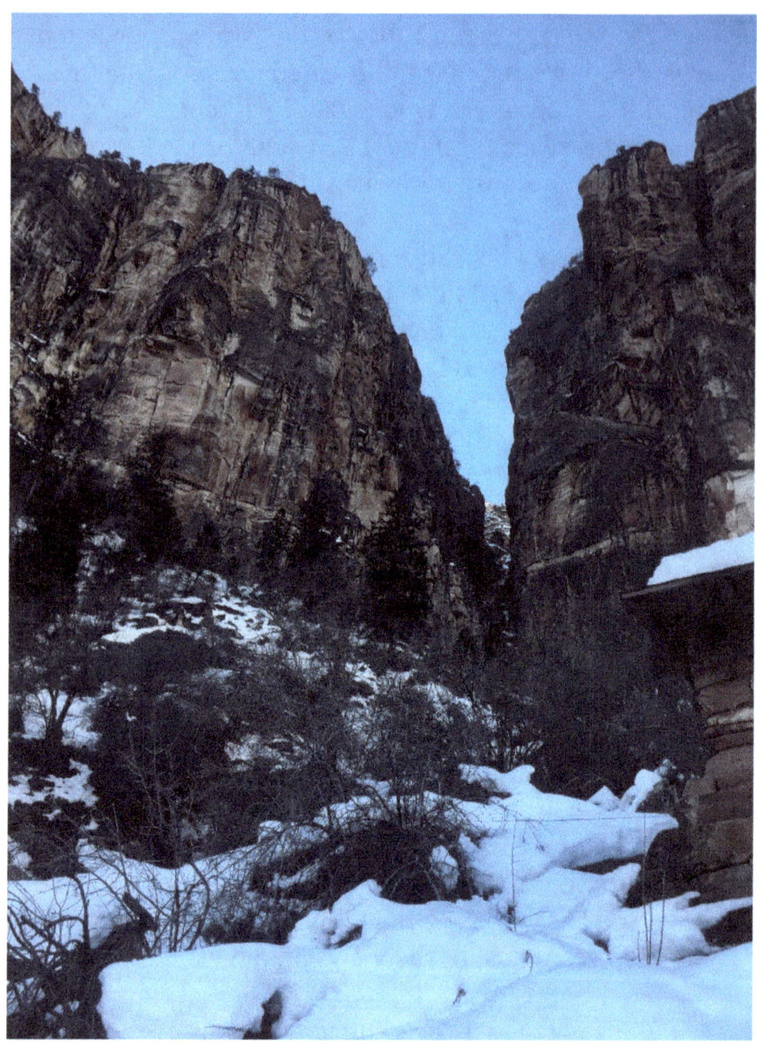

It was inspiring to look back up that canyon wall and think, *"By the end of the day I will be standing on top of that, not even the end of the day 2 pm at most."* By the time 2 pm rolled around I was thinking, *"I've never wanted to push someone off a cliff but if one more person with a selfie stick whacks me their getting an up-close shot of the canyon floor."*

In hindsight I really wish I had used my trekking poles as swords, at least it would have been entertaining.

The thing about the Grand Canyon is your essentially backpacking a mountain in reverse. Most people go up the mountain and then back down, at the Grand Canyon you go down first and then back up. It takes about twice as long to hike up as it took to hike down. I firmly believe at least forty-five minutes of that time is just dealing with traffic jams, usually involving a selfie stick.

I kind of view people the way I view wildlife…from a distance. My job is interacting with people, it's very outgoing and while I love it by the end of the day people just wear you down. It took many years for me to realize I'm an introvert. However, I do like talking to people and helping them out. The amount of people who visit the Grand Canyon made me rethink how people process information, especially in written form. So, for the average day hiker, who only hike a mile or two down, really should pause and read the bulletin boards; especially hiking 101.

"When visiting the Grand Canyon, make sure you hike into the canyon, and be careful not to fall or step in mule poop." – McKenna Shay

BJ's abridged hiking 101 derived from the Grand Canyon site bulletins and informational graphics:

1.  Mules have right away. Don't jump in front of them to take a cool picture, you're holding up the mule train and the rest of the hikers.

2.  Also yelling and jumping because you've seen a mule "in the wild" while said mule is plodding by you, is a great way to scare both the mule and the person riding said mule. Though it's more the rider's reaction to being startled, that effects the mule. It also scares all the hikers who are waiting quietly while the mules pass, especially when the mule decides to jump sideways and almost takes out five people.

3.  Take water. Even though it's February, and the rest houses every mile and a half—have more water that you think. If you're not used to arid conditions (most visitors), you'll need more water. Puking by the side of the trail is not a fun morning activity.

4.  While it's only a "courtesy" on both the website and the bulletin board. Please give the uphill hikers the right of way. You won't realize it until you're coming back up but once you get in a groove of walking, especially uphill, you don't want to stop.

5.  It is a good sign if you can carry a conversation while you're walking and not be out of breath. That said I don't care what you had for lunch last Thursday and when you walk two abreast, I can't pass you. Especially, when you either ignore or didn't hear the "passing on right." Talking is great, however, pay attention to your surroundings. Not

only the other people on the trail there is a whole canyon over there.

6. Please don't wear flip flops. Surprisingly, several people thought this was great footwear. It's February, there is ice on the rim even though it's a desert area. I didn't get to see any broken bones, but odds are high that something might happen.

7. Keep the selfie sticks on the rim—or be selective in how you use them. The trail isn't that wide, in some places, and there are tons of people coming down or up that will be happy to take a photo for you. I got whacked twice by people who were trying to get that perfect shot and weren't paying attention. (I did try to dodge, but when there are people behind, in front, and to the side of you, it's hard to go anywhere.)

Sorry for the rant, but some things bear repeating. Like I said I still enjoyed the hike for the most part. I just would change the time we came back up. I think hiking up at 4 am would have missed most of the people or at least put us near the rim with the first surge of people. Or waiting until about three hours before nightfall.

All in all, though, if you are thinking about taking a backpacking trip into the canyon, weather permitting, February or March is the time to go. Fewer people, pleasant temperatures in the Inner Canyon, and an icy finish.

After plodding along, we reached the mid-point a stone rest house and met up with our driver and hiking companion from the previous day. She brought along another hiker to join our party. We ate a quick lunch. For me that was the other hardboiled egg, a couple of peanut butter bites, and an energy bar.

Two miles later I had the shakes. Not from exhaustion or overexertion but because I wasn't consuming enough calories. I ate the remaining four energy bars and most of the bag of peanut butter bites at a switchback near the top. Our fearless leader felt bad for not catching on that I hadn't eaten enough, I felt like a dumbass because as an EMT and knowledgeable ranger I didn't account for the larger calorie burn.

Craving a cheeseburger, fries, and whole apple pie we resumed the last leg of our journey. It was here I got a little annoyed with some of the members of the group, I'm all for conversation but I was in the "get to the top," eat a burger mindset. I was still in the rear of the group and each time the conversation struck up we would bog down. I started to stop and wait, let them get ahead and catch up.

Once we broached the top of the trail, and dodged the selfie sticks, we on good terms again. I remember stopping at the big bulletin board with large stones, perfect for sitting down and removing crampons. Soon as I had the crampons off, I looked up at the trail head sign for Bright Angel.

I had made it. I survived my first backpacking trip.

I wanted to go again.

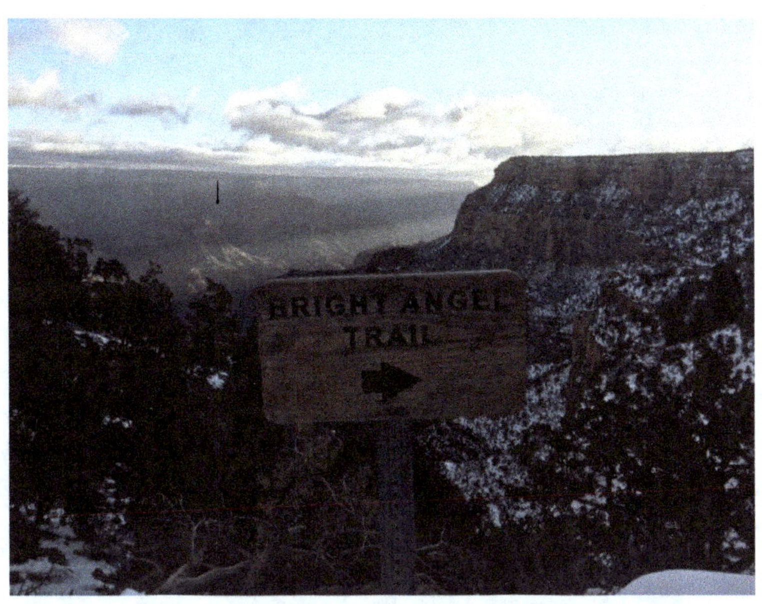
BRIGHT ANGEL
TRAIL

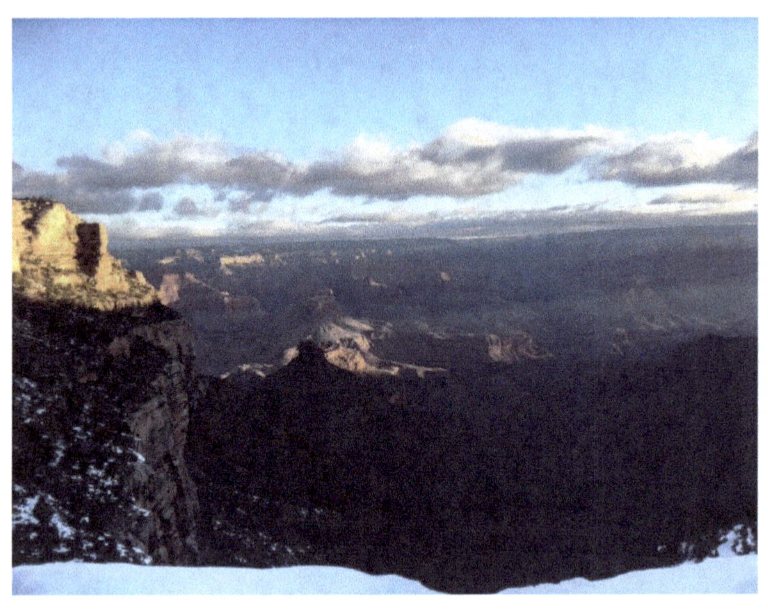

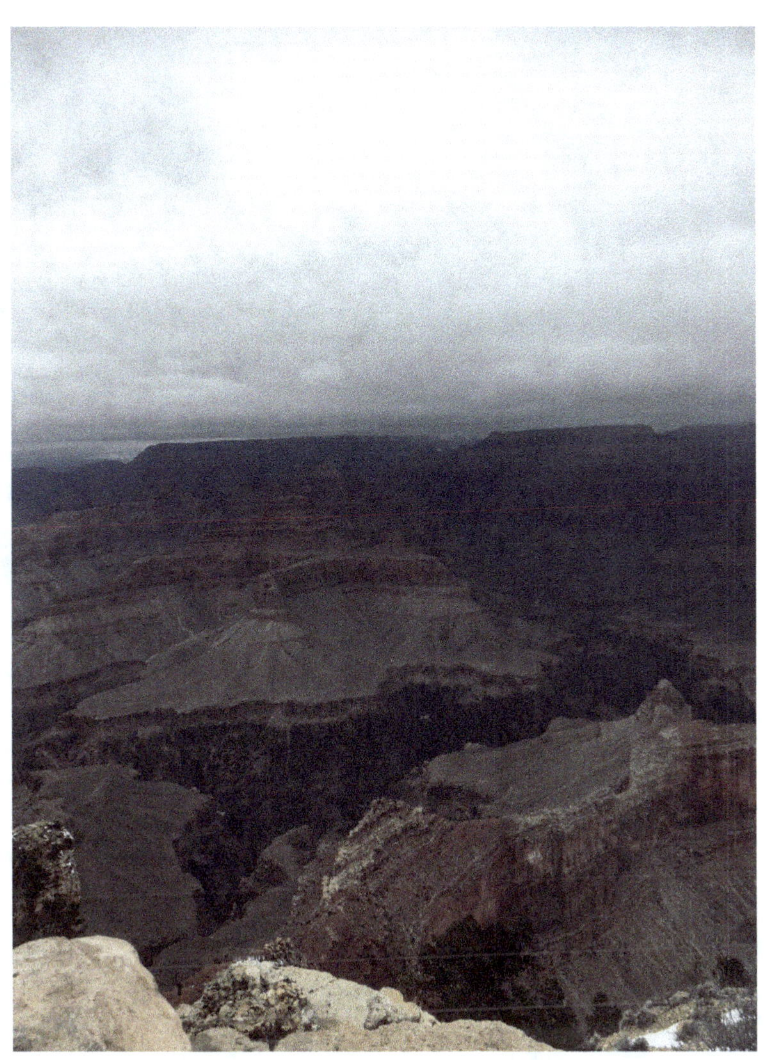

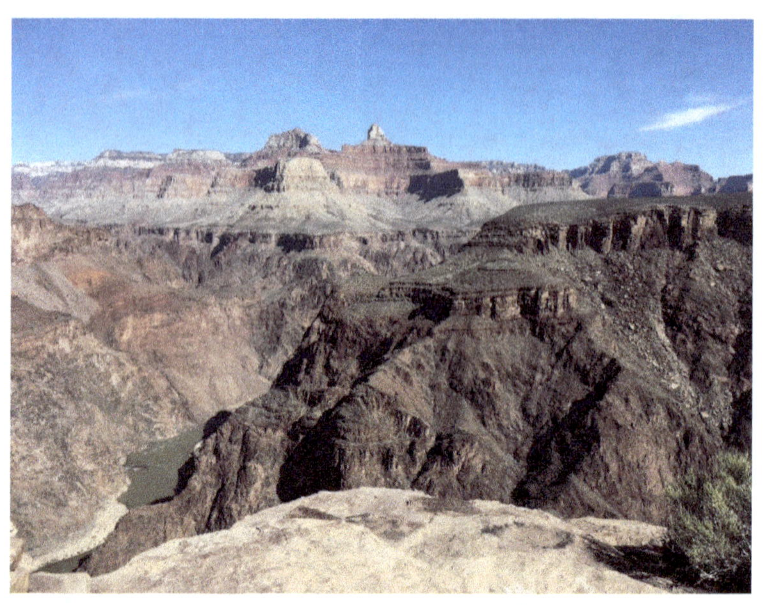

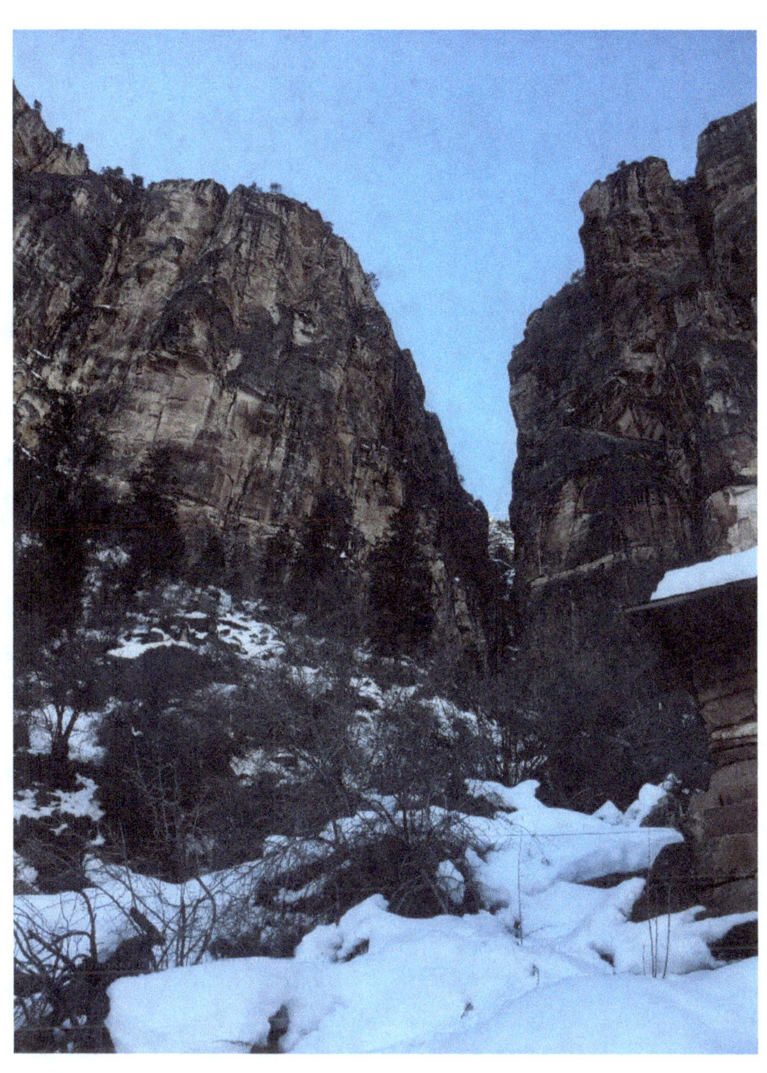

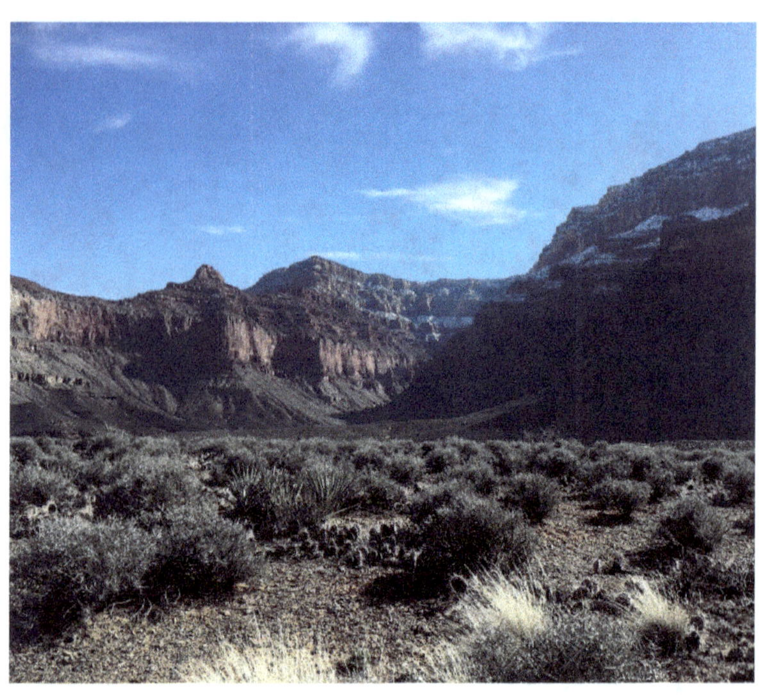

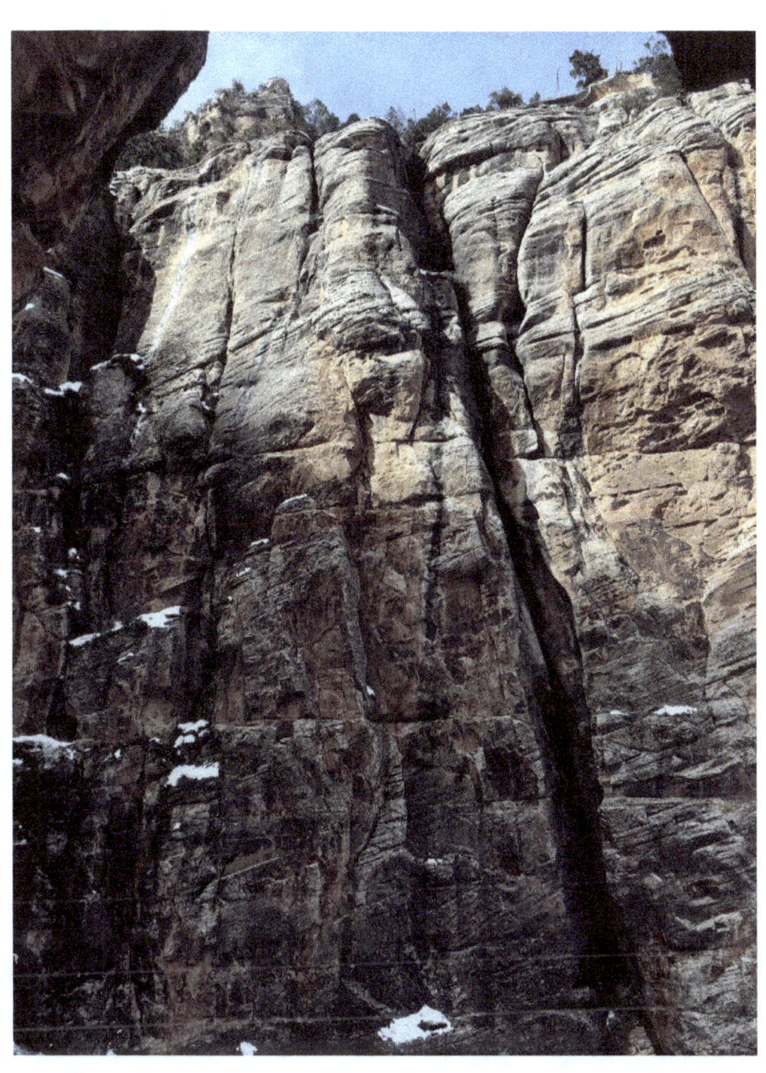

# Part Five: Epilogue

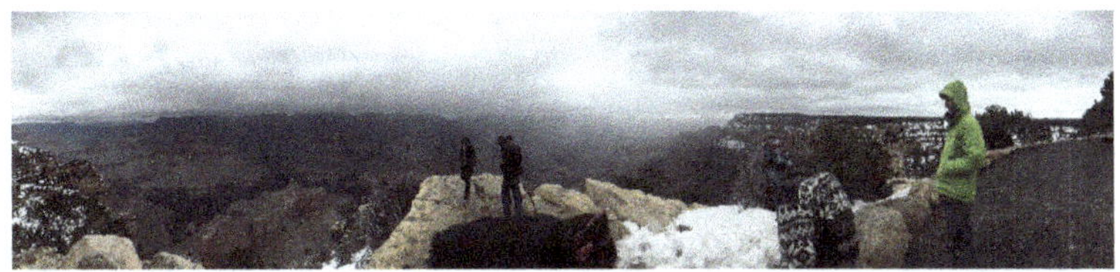

After we finished our trip, the fearless leader and I went and dropped money (in my case a lot of money) in the Grand Canyon Bookstore. Soon as we returned to the lodgings, I ate a quick snack and jumped in the shower. I sighed in pleasure as I lavished each tooth with a healthy dose of toothpaste. Once hygiene had been reestablished, I checked on my online classes. Then I cracked open the first book on my reading list. It was the *Emerald Mile*.

Laying in the bed and reading had a calming effect, i.e. I took an unplanned nap. I awoke to some messages about a Superbowl Party where mass quantities of pizza would be available. I felt like Toot-Toot from the Dresden Files. I hustled down the stairs to the commons. I inhaled a lot of pizza, still recovering from the deficit.

The Superbowl was okay, surprisingly I liked Lady Gaga's halftime show, and I once again fell asleep. This time on the floor. I was awoken by someone who was very excited at the winning team. I groggily made my way back to my room. I still don't recall who won. I was going up the stairs when I felt the first twinges of pain in my calves.

The next day I was sore, but it wasn't too bad, I took my time walking places. It wasn't until Tuesday that the real pain set in. I woke up with a muscle cramp in my left leg. I took a warm bath and that seemed to help. After a long day of training, I was once again heading up those stairs. It was so painful, that I fully implemented a plan for the world's shoddiest rope sling elevator by the time I reached my door.

Unfortunately, I wouldn't be able to realize my plan since I didn't have any rope. A hot bath, two beers, and a couple of low dose pain pills later I was comfortable. I was on the phone with my mom and dad telling them about the trip and the late arriving pain. My mom asked, "Was it worth it?"

Without missing a beat, "Hell Yes!"

I'd do it again in a heartbeat. In fact, I'm trying to convince my fiancée to take a combined rafting/backpacking trip to the Grand Canyon as our honeymoon. He gets to pick the honeymoon since I picked where we're getting married. I keep dropping hints. I'll keep you'll posted.

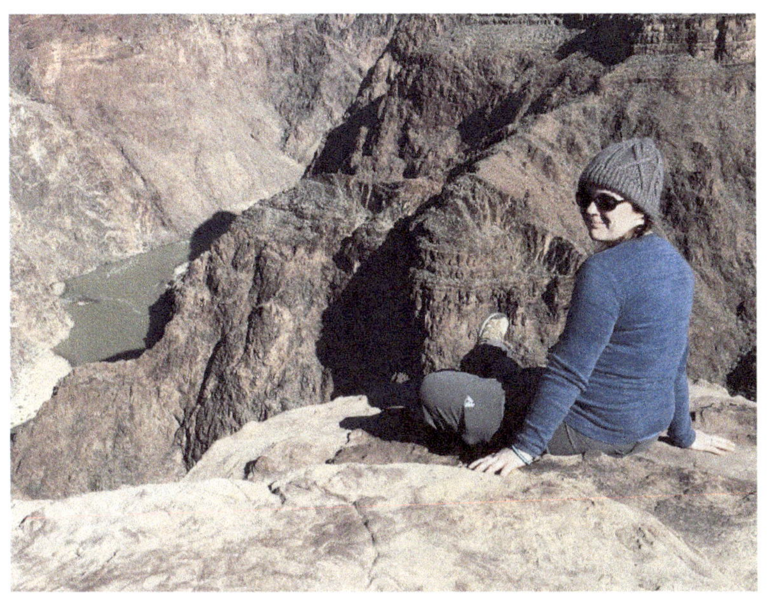

*BJ checking out the Colorado River*
*from Plateau Point*

# BJ's Packing List

While I covered it in the narrative, I wanted to provide a simple list— plus a wish list of items I wished I had.

Backpacking List:

- Modified first aid kit—aside from the standard little first aid kit for bumps and bruises. I tossed in some splitting materials for ankles and wrists. Plus, an extra mylar blanket.
- Crampons or ice cleats.
- Adjustable hiking poles/sticks
- Pack
- Mummy bag
- Mummy bag liner
- Sleeping pad
- Two dry bags
- Two-person tent
- Ground tarp
- Three water bottles (two Smartwater's and a regular Nalgene)
- One Gatorade (I think it was Fruit Punch)
- Four electrolyte packets
- 8 Bumble Bee Tuna Snack Packs
- 10 hardboiled eggs (should have brought 20)
- 5 Cool Mint protein bars
- 5 granola bars
- Peanut butter oatmeal bites
- Contact solution and container.
- Pain pills

- Extra socks and underwear
- Sunglasses case with regular glasses
- Kindle
- New-skin bandages
- Snickers and mini musketeers
- Solar phone charger and cable
- iPhone

Wish List Items:

- Backpacker Pantry meals… all of them.
- MSR backpacking stove—even a little one.
- My backpack—that actually fit me.
- Camelback or other water system with a straw and evenly distributed weight.
- My Canon DSLR or even my Coolpix from Nikon would have sufficed. For my Glacier trip I practiced a carry on to bring my "good" camera.
- Sandals for once I got down below the ice line.
- Midweight jacket or vest.
- My lightweight camp chair.
- My fiancé.
- A selfie stick—the irony I know considering my rant. Once I was down in the canyon and had some alone time it would have been nice to get some shots of me instead of selfies. Plus, I might have been able to get a decent shot of the night sky on my phone—I doubt it but maybe…
- Better iPhone—at the time it was a great phone, but my current iPhone camera is 1,000 times better.

# Recommended Reading List for the Grand Canyon

I love books. I love adventure. I love writing about it. But I love giving book recommendations. When I went to the Grand Canyon I brushed up on a few books—mainly John Wesley Powell's works.

However, I found a plethora of excellent narratives at the Grand Canyon Book Store and had to figure out which ones to buy and figure out how to pack in my carry-on suitcase. While I love physical books—eBooks and my Kindle make traveling, camping, and backpacking so much easier.

Books Recommendations:

- *I Am the Grand Canyon: The Story of the Havasupai People* by Stephen Hirst
- *The Emerald Mile* by Kevin Fedarko
- *The Exploration of the Colorado River and its Canyons* by John Wesley Powell
- *Beyond the Hundredth Meridian: John Wesley Powell and the Second Opening of the West* by Wallace Stegner
- *There's This River… Grand Canyon Boatman Stories* by Christa Sadler
- *Breaking the Current: Boatwomen of the Grand Canyon* by Louise Teal
- *Sunk Without a Sound* by Brad Dimock
- *The Grand Canyon Reader* edited by Lance Newman
- *Canyon* by Michael Ghiglieri
- *Down the River* by Edward Abbey

- *How the Canyon Became Grand: A Short History* by Stephen J. Pyne
- *River Notes: A Natural and Human History of the Colorado* by Wade Davis

# National Park Service Hiking Tips for the Grand Canyon

I wanted to make sure people had access to an all-in-one spot to find this information.

Here is the website: [Hiking Tips - Hike Smart - Grand Canyon National Park (U.S. National Park Service) (nps.gov)](nps.gov)

Plus, here are a few highlights for hiking I think everyone should know!

- Be lightweight—don't overpack.
- If you're huffing and puffing, you're not getting enough oxygen. Be able to walk and talk comfortably.
- (Relevant for me) No Food, No Fuel, No Fun
- If you're hiking in summer, plan around shade—hang out between 10 am and 4 pm.
- Building on the previous, flop in the water to get soaked and hike yourself dry. It will help you stay cool.
- Drink to ease thirst, not to guzzle. If you drink to much you through off your electrolyte. Between that and the dry air you will sweat off and flush away your salt and cause hyponatremia… so bring your electrolyte powder and drink slowly.
- Winter hiking—wear layers and traction for ice
- Sunblock. Just have it no matter the time of year.

# Reflections

Thanks for reading this abridged version of my blog post. I hope to create series based off some of my more extensive hikes in the future.

Looking back this adventure to the Grand Canyon was a defining moment for me. I'm still trying to recreate the magic of that trip and the inspiration for writing. My blog is hit or miss—life is keeping me pretty busy and it's hard to get out and create situations to write about. It's gone through a few iterations now—hiking, to hiking books (thanks Covid), to hiking with kids, to being kind of like a personal journal I'm still trying.

Yet, that hike into the canyon awakened me and I'm hoping to introduce my kids to nature and beautiful places will get me back out there again.

Also, we wound up going on a Caribbean Cruise for our honeymoon but I'm thinking for our 2027 anniversary we go to the Grand Canyon. Until then—Keep Wandering.

- BJ the Wannabe Backpacker
10/26/2023

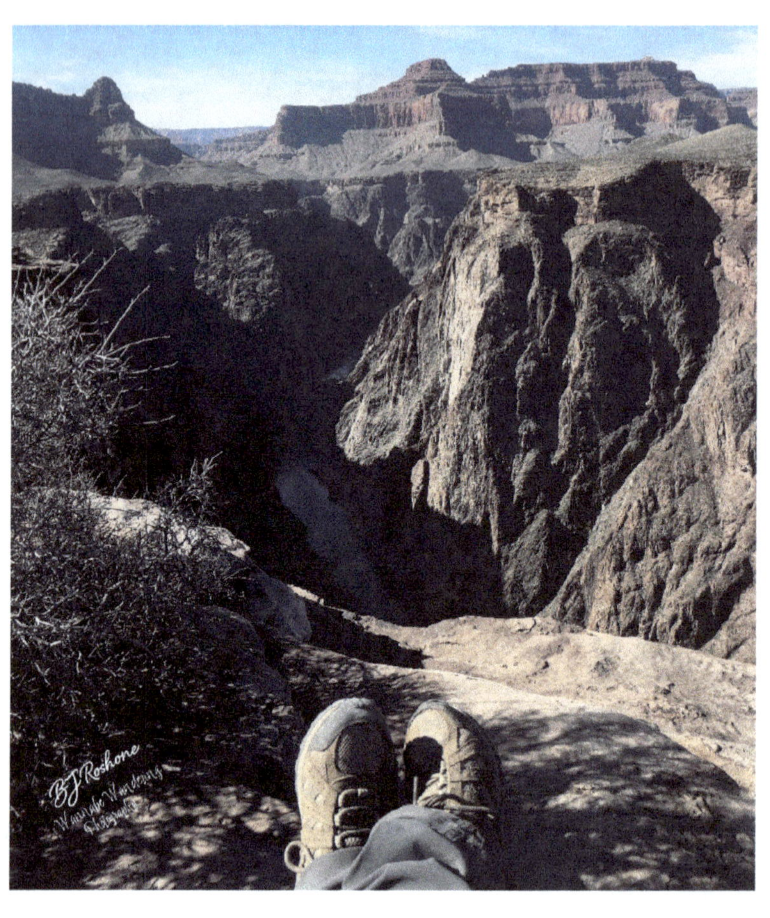
BJ Roshone
Wannabe Wandering
Photography

www.ingramcontent.com/pod-product-compliance
Lightning Source LLC
Chambersburg PA
CBHW050847260726

48660CB00006B/2498